Lectin Free Slow Cooker Cookbook

Quick and Easy Lectin Free Slow Cooker Recipes

Mellisa Armstrong
Copyright © 2018 Mellisa Armstrong
All rights reserved.

TABLE OF CONTENTS

1	What are Lectins?	4
2	What's Wrong with Lectins?	5
3	Foods Recommended Eating	7
4	Foods Recommended Avoiding	9
5	Lectin-Free Diet and Its Benefits	10
6	Lectin-Free Breakfast Recipes using Crock-Pot	11
7	Lectin-Free Poultry Recipes using Crock-Pot	31
8	Lectin-Free Seafood Recipes using Crock-Pot	51
9	Lectin-Free Beef, Pork and Lamb using Crock-Pot	72
10	About the Author	93

COPYRIGHT 2018 BY MELLISA ARMSTRONG - ALL RIGHTS RESERVED.

This document is geared towards providing exact and reliable information in regard to the topic and issue covered. The publication is sold on the idea that the publisher is not required to render an accounting, officially permitted, or otherwise, qualified services. If advice is necessary, legal or professional, a practised individual in the profession should be ordered.

From a Declaration of Principles which was accepted and approved equally by a Committee of the American Bar Association and a Committee of Publishers and Associations.

In no way is it legal to reproduce, duplicate, or transmit any part of this document by either electronic means or in printed format. Recording of this publication is strictly prohibited and any storage of this document is not allowed unless with written permission from the publisher. All rights reserved.

The information provided herein is stated to be truthful and consistent, in that any liability, in terms of inattention or otherwise, by any usage or abuse of any policies, processes, or directions contained within is the solitary and utter responsibility of the recipient reader. Under no circumstances will any legal responsibility or blame be held against the publisher for any reparation, damages, or monetary loss due to the information herein, either directly or indirectly.

Respective authors own all copyrights not held by the publisher. The information herein is offered for informational purposes solely and is universal as so. The presentation of the information is without a contract or any type of guarantee assurance.

The trademarks that are used are without any consent, and the publication of the trademark is without permission or backing by the trademark owner. All trademarks and brands within this book are for clarifying purposes only and are the owned by the owners themselves, not affiliated with this document.

WHAT ARE LECTINS?

As a kind of protein, lectins work as a defense system in plants. Experts believe that plants use these proteins to save themselves from insects. Scientifically, the function of lectins includes the binding process of carbohydrates.

In humans, lectins possibly help with an interactive activity in cells. The construction of lectin proteins includes nitrogen. Plants use this component to ensure their growth. Hence, there are various plant parts that contain lectins. However, humans eat only one of those parts, i.e., seed.

It is possible that lectins create certain health changes in one's body. The effects can be diverse such as digestion issues, cluster of blood cells, and even chronic diseases. These proteins also stop the body from utilizing certain nutrients. That is why many experts categorize this component as antinutrients.

If eaten uncooked, many plant foods can create digestion issues. This also happens due to the high consistency of lectins. Your stomach can even get disturbed if a plant food is not cooked properly.

The red beans, also known as kidney beans, contain a special kind of lectin. This lectin is known as phytohaemagglutinin. This component causes the bean poisoning in people who eat undercooked red beans.

WHAT'S WRONG WITH LECTINS?

As mentioned earlier, many experts consider lectins as antinutrients. Their ability to restrict the nutrients' absorption makes them highly risky for the human body. Also, it possibly comes into the category of inflammatory toxins too. Hence, they induce the problem of weight gain. It starts with digestive issues, which can also lead to brain fog, acne, arthritis, and various other issues.

Even a little amount of phytohaemagglutinin can cause digestive problems. Thankfully, lectins become inactive with proper cooking. It all comes down to keeping the temperature high. That is why using pressure cooking is preferred for red beans.

However, the lectin content is not just limited to seeds. There are various food components that give you lectins:

- GRAINS: It would not be wrong to say that grains are the last plant-based food discovery for humans. In ancient times, humans never tried to find grains in their searches. Almost all types of grains come with a vast availability of lectin. Even the gluten-free choices of grains give a lot of lectin to the body. Hence, it is better to restrict the number of grains you intake. One great change would be shifting to white flour from wheat flour.

- LEGUMES AND BEANS: Beans contain the maximum quantity of lectins. Lentils, peas, beans, and all other legumes come under this category. Experts suggest pressure cooking for these legumes to remove the lectins properly. Eating cashews and peanuts can increase lectins in your body too. So, avoid these two if possible.

- SQUASH: Every vegetable that contains seeds comes under fruit category. As you already know, seeds are the storage point of lectins in plants. Hence, squash, zucchini, pumpkins, and other seed-containing veggies are a big no for you. If you need the nutrients of squash, get rid of the seeds and peels before cooking.

- CERTAIN FRUITS: Various fruits such as grapes, pomegranate, and other seed-containing fruits give you lectins. However, you can enjoy these fruits if they are in season. But make sure that you include them in your diet in a limited quantity.

- NIGHTSHADE VEGETABLES: In the nightshade category, you have to worry about lectins too. Vegetables such as eggplant, tomatoes, potatoes, and all kinds of pepper come within this category. The seeds and the peels store too much lectins. That is why one needs to remove seeds and avoid peels. Then, properly cook in a pressure cooker or an Instant Pot to diminish the lectin quantity. Experts also suggest fermentation process to make these vegetables lectin free.

Lectins are especially risky for humans due to the unavailability of proper enzymes. The human body doesn't contain the required enzymes to actually digest these proteins. Hence, lectins don't change much in terms of structure in our digestive system. That is why regular intake can generate a layer of lectins in the intestines. This layer limits the nutrient absorption capacity of the intestines. In fact, the digestive tract changes its functionality due to the change in available space.

All these problems lead to leaky gut problems, autoimmune diseases, and other issues. The person can lose control of his or her gut. Then, lectins can also reach blood cells and attack antibodies. This directly reduces the immunity in a person, making the cells damaged and weak. Similar autoimmune issues are related to the lectin proteins that are available in tomatoes.

FOODS RECOMMENDED EATING

Apart from cooking your food properly, you can also divert your diet to certain food choices in order to avoid lectins:

LEAFY GREENS: To avoid lectin, one can shift his or her diet toward lettuce, romaine, spinach, mesclun, parsley, butter lettuce, fennel, and sea veggies as well. These leafy greens provide required nutrients to the body without presenting the risks of lectins.

TUBERS AFTER COOKING: Tubers such as taro root and sweet potatoes are highly effective to receive minerals and vitamins. Being a root, such vegetables provide proper water and other minerals to the body. However, it is extremely important to cook them at a high temperature properly.

CRUCIFEROUS VEGETABLES: With cauliflower, broccoli, and even brussels sprouts, one can get the required nourishment without taking lectins. All the cruciferous veggies are perfect to reduce the lectin amount and receive quality nourishment on a daily basis.

MUSHROOMS: Mushrooms are a great source of fiber as well as polyphenols. You can include different kinds of mushrooms such as cremini and others in your diet. These mushrooms also go well with different pork, beef, and lamb recipes. That is why you can replace lectin-rich vegetables with mushrooms and make your recipes lectin free.

CELERY: For high fiber, you should also include celery in your diet. Celery provides polyphenols and doesn't contain lectins. Hence, including this ingredient in your diet will be safe for a lectin-free diet.

GARLIC AND ONION: These two are also on the green side of the lectin-free ingredients.

AVOCADO: This fruit is known for its antioxidant powers. However, avocado is usable in your diet if ripe. The fruit contains no sugar. It provides a high amount of soluble fiber as well as good fat. Hence, people looking for weight loss should use avocado in their diet for sure.

OLIVE OIL: Shifting to olive oil is the prime requirement to avoid the lectins that reach your body through other cooking oils. Prefer extra-virgin oil of olives, but you can work with natural olive oil as well. This oil is a direct source of minerals and vitamins. A variety of nutritional properties such as vitamin E, vitamin K, sodium, iron, calcium, and even potassium are a part of olive oil. The fatty acids content makes this oil an essential addition to your lectin-free diet. According to experts, olive oil has the capacity to reduce the inflammatory actions in your body that lead to autoimmune disorders.

A2 MILK: The milk that contains A2 type of proteins only provides a lectin-free dairy option. These kinds of milk provide all types of essential nutritional values such as magnesium, potassium, phosphorus, zinc, various vitamins, and others. By providing the A2 type of protein, this milk saves from lectins. Hence, you can include this type of milk in your diet.

Finally, here is an overview of what you should include in your lectin-free diet:

- Sweet potatoes, properly cooked
- Meats that are pasture-raised
- Green vegetables that majorly contain leafy texture
- A2 milk
- Asparagus
- Cruciferous vegetables (for example, brussels sprouts, broccoli, etc.)
- Celery
- Onion
- Mushrooms
- Garlic
- Olives
- Avocado
- Olive oil

FOODS RECOMMENDED AVOIDING

Certain food options are a big no if you want to avoid lectins:

CORN-FED MEATS: Corns are full of lectins, which is why the same lectins reach the animals that eat them. Corn-fed lamb, pork, chicken, and even eggs are a big NO for you. The deposits of lectins increase with such meat. Hence, you need to shift toward pasture-fed meat that comes from the animals that eat grass in their diet.

A1 MILK: The A1 protein in cow's milk is a result of mutation. A1 protein has similar effects on humans as the lectins do. The mutation happened in the cows from Northern Europe. This genetic mutation has created A1 casein protein that harms the pancreas. Hence, your goal should be to avoid all dairy products that include A1 milk. These products can be heavy cream, cheese, milk, and others. Instead, choose dairy products that are prepared from the A2 milk.

Here is a quick list of all the food choices one should avoid in order to maintain a safe distance from lectins:

- Squash
- Peas
- Beans
- Lentils
- Eggplant
- Potatoes
- Tomatoes
- Peppers
- Grains
- Meat yield from animals that are corn-fed
- Corn
- A1 milk

LECTIN-FREE DIET AND ITS BENEFITS

When you decide to go lectin-free, it removes certain foods from your diet. Legumes, grains, quinoa, and even those nightshade vegetables have to go out of your kitchen. Along with that, you need to become careful about the meat selection and dairy products too.

A lectin-free diet focuses on leafy vegetables. Your veggie selections move toward options such as broccoli, cauliflower, mushrooms, and asparagus. In terms of meat selection, you choose meats that are pasture-raised. Also, the fish options become limited to wild-caught.

With a disciplined approach, one can improve his or her health and also lose some unnecessary weight. Such a diet also helps in improving your body from metabolic syndrome. Your body maintains a balance of blood sugars and blood pressure.

There are various benefits that experts associate with a lectin-free diet:

- SAFETY FROM INFLAMMATION

Inflammation is a direct problem that lectins create in your body. Lectin-free diet saves the intestines from the accumulation of undigested lectin layers. Hence, the digestive tract stays clear. This saves from inflammation and digestive issues as well. The same inflammation presents the risk of heart diseases and even depression. Some experts also connect lectin intake with cancer. Hence, a lectin-free diet seems like a wise choice for any person.

- HELPS LOSING WEIGHT

The limited diet option becomes a great help in achieving your weight loss goals. A lectin-free diet diverts you toward leafy vegetables, olive oil, and other nutrition friendly choices. Plus, your body doesn't receive lectins that disturb the metabolic system. Hence, your body naturally loses weight.

The benefits of a lectin-free diet depend immensely on the discipline you apply. Various food options go out of the list, which requires proper planning. Otherwise, your body can feel the lack of various nutrients. Hence, you need a set weekly plan to manage nutrition intake.

LECTIN-FREE BREAKFAST RECIPES USING CROCK-POT

VEGGIE OMELET

SERVING SIZE: 1
SERVINGS PER RECIPE: 4
CALORIES: 142
COOKING TIME: 2 HOURS 10 MINUTES

INGREDIENTS:

Eggs—6

Milk—½ cup

Salt—¼ teaspoon

Fresh ground pepper—to taste

Garlic powder—1/8 teaspoon or to taste

Chili powder—1/8 teaspoon or to taste

Broccoli florets—1 cup

Yellow onion—1, small, finely chopped

Garlic clove—1, minced

Shredded cheddar cheese—for garnishing

Chopped onions—for garnishing

Fresh parsley—for garnishing

NUTRITION INFORMATION:

Carbohydrate—8g

Protein—10 g

Fat—7 g

Sodium—263 mg

Cholesterol—248 mg

INSTRUCTIONS:

1. Take a Crock-Pot and lightly grease the inside of it with cooking spray. Set it aside.

2. Take a large mixing bowl and crack six eggs into it. Combine the eggs with milk, salt, pepper, garlic powder, and chili powder. Mix it well by using a whisk or an eggbeater to combine the mixture well.

3. In the Crock-Pot, add in broccoli florets, garlic, and onion. Pour in the egg mixture into it.

4. Cover the Crock-Pot and cook for about 2 hours on high heat. When the eggs set, the omelet is ready.

5. Sprinkle some cheese on top and cover the lid for about 2–3 minutes to allow the cheese to melt.

6. Cut the omelet into four wedges. Place the omelet on a plate.

7. Sprinkle some chopped onions and fresh parsley for garnishing.

8. Your veggie omelet is ready to be served.

FRENCH TOAST CASSEROLE WITH NUTELLA AND CARAMELIZED BANANAS

SERVING SIZE: 1
SERVINGS PER RECIPE: 8
CALORIES: 150
COOKING TIME: 2 HOURS 15 MINUTES

INGREDIENTS:

- Barley bread—1 lb., grain-free, cut into cubes
- Large eggs—6
- Vanilla almond milk—2 cups
- Ground cinnamon—1 teaspoon
- Vanilla extract—1 tablespoon
- Nutella—2 tablespoons plus some for topping
- Salt—to taste
- Unsalted butter—1 tablespoon
- Bananas—4, sliced
- Brown sugar—1 tablespoon

NUTRITION INFORMATION:

- Carbohydrate—18 g
- Protein—6 g
- Fat—7 g
- Sodium—90 mg
- Cholesterol—160 mg

INSTRUCTIONS:

1. Take the Crock-Pot and place cubes of bread into it.

2. Take a large bowl and add eggs, milk, vanilla extract, and cinnamon to it. Add in Nutella and salt and whisk it well to combine the mixture.

3. Pour in the mixture over the cubes of bread into the Crock-Pot. Mix it well to coat the bread cubes completely.

4. Cover the lid of the Crock-Pot and let it cook for 2 hours on high heat.

5. Add some sliced bananas to a bowl. Add in the brown sugar with the banana and mix well.

6. Take a sauté pan and add butter to it at medium-high heat. Put the banana slices in the butter in the pan. Allow it to cook for 2 minutes on each side until they turn brown in color.

7. Take a spoonful of the French toast mixture from the Crock-Pot and top it with caramelized banana.

8. Add an extra spoon of Nutella as garnish.

9. Your dish is ready to be served.

SPINACH AND MOZZARELLA FRITTATA

SERVING SIZE: 1
SERVINGS PER RECIPE: 6
CALORIES: 139
COOKING TIME: 1 HOUR 45 MINUTES

INGREDIENTS:

- Extra-virgin olive oil—1 tablespoon
- Diced onion—½ cup
- Mozzarella cheese—1 cup, divided, shredded
- Eggs—3
- Egg whites—3
- Milk—2 tablespoons
- Black pepper—¼ teaspoon
- White pepper—¼ teaspoon
- Baby spinach—1 cup, chopped, stems removed
- Salt—to taste

NUTRITION INFORMATION:

- Carbohydrate—4 g
- Protein—12 g
- Fat—8 g
- Sodium—mg
- Cholesterol—94 mg

INSTRUCTIONS:

1. Take a small skillet and heat up some oil in it. Add onions in it. Cook the onions for about 5 minutes on medium heat until they become tender.

2. Grease the inside of the Crock-Pot with a nonstick cooking spray.

3. Take a large bowl and combine the eggs, sautéed onion with ¾ cup of mozzarella cheese, and remaining ingredients. Combine the mixture by whisking it well and pour it into the Crock-Pot.

4. Add in the remaining ¼ cup of cheese on the egg mixture.

5. Cover the lid of the Crock-Pot and allow it to cook for 1 ½ hours on low heat until the eggs are completely done.

6. Cut it up into six pieces and serve them.

TURKEY BREAKFAST CASSEROLE

SERVING SIZE: 1
SERVINGS PER RECIPE: 8
CALORIES: 453
COOKING TIME: 6 HOURS 30 MINUTES

INGREDIENTS:

- Mashed sweet potato—30 oz., boiled
- Turkey breakfast sausage—1 lb., cooked, drained
- Yellow onion—1, chopped
- Colby Jack cheese—2 cups, shredded
- Eggs—1 dozen
- Milk—1 cup
- Flour—4 tablespoons
- Salt—1 teaspoon
- Pepper—½ teaspoon
- Crushed red pepper flakes—½ teaspoon

NUTRITION INFORMATION:

- Carbohydrate—28 g
- Protein—25 g
- Fat—9 g
- Sodium—709 mg
- Cholesterol—71 mg

INSTRUCTIONS:

1. In a large bowl, mix the mashed sweet potato with butter, salt, and pepper.

2. Take the Crock-Pot and grease it well. Add a layer of $1/3^{rd}$ of the mashed sweet potato, followed by a layer of turkey sausage. Then goes in the layer of onions and then cheese. Repeat this process twice.

3. Whisk together all the remaining ingredients in a large bowl. Pour the mixture into the Crock-Pot.

4. Cover the lid of the Crock-Pot and allow it to cook for about 6–8 hours on low heat.

5. Your Turkey breakfast casserole is ready to be served.

GREEK EGGS BREAKFAST CASSEROLE

SERVING SIZE: 1
SERVINGS PER RECIPE: 4
CALORIES: 305
COOKING TIME: 4 HOURS

INGREDIENTS:

- Eggs—12, whisked
- Milk—½ cup
- Salt—½ teaspoon
- Black pepper—1 teaspoon
- Red onion—1 tablespoon
- Garlic—1 teaspoon
- Sun-dried tomato—½ cup
- Baby bella mushrooms—1 cup, sliced
- Spinach—2 cups
- Feta cheese—½ cup

NUTRITION INFORMATION:

- Carbohydrate—8 g
- Protein—23 g
- Fat—20 g
- Sodium—378 mg
- Cholesterol—358 mg

INSTRUCTIONS:

1. Take a large mixing bowl and whisk the eggs along with milk, salt, and pepper. Add in the red onions and garlic to the mixture.

2. Combine the sun-dried tomatoes, mushrooms, and spinach to the mixture.

3. Take the Crock-Pot and put the mixture into it. Sprinkle feta cheese on top of it.

4. Allow it to cook for about 4–6 hours on low heat.

5. Your dish is ready to be served.

PEANUT BUTTER BANANA OATMEAL

SERVING SIZE: 1
SERVINGS PER RECIPE: 6
CALORIES: 244
COOKING TIME: 7 HOURS

INGREDIENTS:

- Ripe bananas—2, mashed
- Peanut butter—¼ cup
- Milk—3 cups
- Brown sugar blend—3 tablespoons
- Cinnamon—1 teaspoon
- Vanilla—1 teaspoon
- Steel-cut oatmeal—1 cup
- Bananas—for topping
- Brown sugar blend—for topping

NUTRITION INFORMATION:

- Carbohydrate—33 g
- Protein—7 g
- Fat—6 g
- Sodium—63 mg
- Cholesterol—2 mg

INSTRUCTIONS:

1. Take a medium bowl and add mashed bananas and peanut butter in it. With a hand mixer, blend it well. Now add milk, cinnamon, brown sugar, and vanilla into it. Mix it well.

2. Add the oatmeal into the mixture.

3. Place the bowl of oatmeal mixture in the Crock-Pot. Add about 1 inch of water below the bowl's rim. Cover the lid of the Crock-Pot and allow it to cook on low heat for about 7–8 hours.

4. Remove the bowl from the Crock-Pot. Stir well to combine the mixture.

5. Garnish it with bananas and brown sugar blend.

6. Your oatmeal is ready to be served.

CARAMEL APPLE ROLLS

SERVING SIZE: 1
SERVINGS PER RECIPE: 8
CALORIES: 458
COOKING TIME: 2 HOURS 30 MINUTES

INGREDIENTS:

- Cinnamon rolls with caramel icing—13 oz., cut into 1-inch pieces
- Apples—2, peeled, diced
- Eggs—4
- Heavy cream—½ cup
- Brown sugar—¼ cup
- Vanilla—2 teaspoons
- Cinnamon—1 teaspoon

NUTRITION INFORMATION:

- Carbohydrate—47 g
- Protein—2 g
- Fat—6 g
- Sodium—404 mg
- Cholesterol—1 mg

INSTRUCTIONS:

1. Grease the inside of the Crock-Pot with a nonstick cooking spray.

2. Take half of the cinnamon rolls and place it at the bottom of the Crock-Pot. Add diced apples on top of it.

3. In a small bowl, add eggs, brown sugar, cinnamon, cream, and vanilla. Pour this mixture on top of the layer of the cinnamon rolls. Place the remaining cinnamon rolls on top of this.

4. Pour some of the caramel icings on the top of the layer of the cinnamon rolls.

5. Allow it to cook on low heat for about 2 ½–3 hours until the cinnamon rolls are well cooked. Pour the remaining caramel icing over the cinnamon rolls.

6. Your caramel apple rolls are ready to be served.

EGG, SPINACH, AND HAM BREAKFAST CASSEROLE

SERVING SIZE: 1
SERVINGS PER RECIPE: 6
CALORIES: 126
COOKING TIME: 1 HOUR 30 MINUTES

INGREDIENTS:

- Eggs—6, large
- Salt—½ teaspoon
- Black pepper—¼ teaspoon
- Milk—¼ cup
- Greek yogurt—½ cup
- Thyme—½ teaspoon
- Onion powder—½ teaspoon
- Garlic powder—½ teaspoon
- Mushrooms—1/3 cup, diced
- Baby spinach—1 cup
- Pepper Jack cheese—1 cup, shredded
- Ham—1 cup, diced

NUTRITION INFORMATION:

- Carbohydrate—6 g
- Protein—14 g
- Fat—2 g
- Sodium—1150 mg
- Cholesterol—4.7 mg

INSTRUCTIONS:

1. Take a bowl and add eggs, thyme, onion powder, garlic powder, salt, pepper, milk, and yogurt in it. Mix it well until smooth.

2. Add in the mushrooms, cheese, ham, and spinach.

3. Grease the inside of the Crock-Pot with a nonstick cooking spray.

4. Pour the eggs mixture into the Crock-Pot.

5. Cover the lid of the Crock-Pot and allow it to cook on high heat for about 90 minutes until the eggs are completely set.

6. Slice it evenly and serve.

PEACH OATMEAL

SERVING SIZE: 1
SERVINGS PER RECIPE: 2
CALORIES: 130
COOKING TIME: 4 HOURS

INGREDIENTS:

    Milk—2 cups

    Old-fashioned oats—1 cup, dry

    Peaches in light syrup—1 cup, diced

    Brown sugar—2 tablespoons

    Light butter spread—1 tablespoon

    Honey—2 tablespoons

    Cinnamon—½ teaspoon

    Salt—¼ teaspoon

NUTRITION INFORMATION:

    Carbohydrate—27 g

    Protein—3 g

    Fat—2 g

    Sodium—180 mg

    Cholesterol—0 mg

INSTRUCTIONS:

1. Take a medium bowl and add all the ingredients to it. Mix it together.

2. Grease the inside of the Crock-Pot with a cooking spray. Pour the oatmeal mixture into the Crock-Pot. Cover the lid of the Crock-Pot and allow it to cook on low heat for about 4 hours.

3. Make sure the oats turn soft when finished.

4. Pour milk on top of the oats.

5. Your peach oatmeal is ready to be served.

THREE CHEESE SHRIMP AND GRITS

SERVING SIZE: 1
SERVINGS PER RECIPE: 8
CALORIES: 484
COOKING TIME: 3 HOURS 30 MINUTES

INGREDIENTS:

- Chicken broth—6 cups
- Quick cooking grits—1 ½ cups
- Garlic powder—1 tablespoon
- Onion powder—1 tablespoon
- Dried thyme—1 teaspoon
- Salt—to taste
- Pepper—to taste
- Cheddar cheese—1 cup
- Light cream cheese—4 oz.
- Parmesan—½ cup, grated
- Hot sauce—½ teaspoon
- Raw shrimp—2 pounds
- Scallions—for garnishing
- Parmesan cheese—for garnishing

NUTRITION INFORMATION:

- Carbohydrate—47 g
- Protein—25 g
- Fat—21 g
- Sodium—1232 mg
- Cholesterol—137 mg

INSTRUCTIONS:

1. Take the Crock-Pot and add grits and chicken broth in it. Then add all the other ingredients except green onions and shrimp.

2. Allow it to cook on low heat for about 3 hours.

3. Add the shrimp into the Crock-Pot. Cook for another 30 minutes until the shrimps turn pink and are cooked thoroughly.

4. Garnish it with chopped green onions. Sprinkle grated parmesan cheese.

5. Your dish is ready to be served.

LECTIN-FREE POULTRY RECIPES USING CROCK-POT

CHICKEN PARMESAN

SERVING SIZE: 1
SERVINGS PER RECIPE: 8
CALORIES: 1166
COOKING TIME: 5 HOURS 40 MINUTES

INGREDIENTS:

- Vegetable oil—2 tablespoons
- Chicken breast halves—8, boneless
- Salt—to taste
- Pepper—to taste
- Italian seasoning—as needed
- Spaghetti sauce—2 cups
- Bay leaf—1
- Garlic powder—as desired
- Mozzarella cheese—1 cup, shredded
- Parmesan cheese—for garnishing
- Cooked noodles—12 oz.

NUTRITION INFORMATION:

- Carbohydrate—43 g
- Protein—109 g
- Fat—59 g
- Sodium—395 mg
- Cholesterol—321 mg

INSTRUCTIONS:

1. Take a large skillet and heat oil in it over medium heat. Add the chicken in the skillet and allow it to brown well. Season it with salt, pepper, and Italian seasoning as required.

2. Take the Crock-Pot and put bay leaf, garlic, and spaghetti sauce in it. Combine them well. Place the chicken in the sauce and cover the lid of the Crock-Pot. Allow it to cook on low heat for about 5–6 hours. The chicken should be thoroughly cooked through and soft.

3. Transfer the chicken to a casserole dish. Pour the sauce all over it. Sprinkle both mozzarella and parmesan cheese on top of it. Allow it to heat at 350°F until the cheese has completely melted.

4. Place the noodles on a plate. Pour the chicken along with the sauce over it.

5. Your chicken parmesan is ready to be served.

ISLAND BARBECUED TURKEY LEGS

SERVING SIZE: 1
SERVINGS PER RECIPE: 6
CALORIES: 2479
COOKING TIME: 7 HOURS

INGREDIENTS:

    Turkey legs—6

    Kosher salt—to taste

    Freshly ground black pepper—to taste

    Cider vinegar—5 tablespoons

    Worcestershire sauce—1 tablespoon

    Dark brown sugar—4 tablespoons

    Liquid smoke—1 teaspoon

    Pineapple—8 oz., 1 can, crushed, well drained

    Onion—½ cup, chopped

NUTRITION INFORMATION:

    Carbohydrate—24 g

    Protein—363 g

    Fat—94 g

    Sodium—2244 mg

    Cholesterol—1206 mg

INSTRUCTIONS:

1. Spray the inside of the Crock-Pot with cooking spray.

2. Place the turkey legs in the Crock-Pot and season it with salt and pepper.

3. Take a bowl and add all the remaining ingredients in it. Coat the turkey legs well with the mixture.

4. Cover the lid of the Crock-Pot and allow it to cook on low heat for about 7 hours until tender.

5. Your dish is ready to be served.

TURKEY STROGANOFF

SERVING SIZE: 1
SERVINGS PER RECIPE: 5
CALORIES: 235
COOKING TIME: 5 HOURS

INGREDIENTS:

Lean ground turkey—1 lb.

Onion—1, diced

Button mushrooms—4 oz., sliced

Chicken broth—1 cup, low sodium, fat-free

Balsamic vinegar—1 tablespoon

Black pepper—½ teaspoon

Salt—to taste

Greek yogurt—1 cup, low fat

Cornstarch—2 tablespoons

NUTRITION INFORMATION:

Carbohydrate—17 g

Protein—21 g

Fat—9 g

Sodium—252 mg

Cholesterol—71 mg

INSTRUCTIONS:

1. Take a large skillet and put ground turkey in it. Cook until it is no longer pink in color. Drain off the excess fat from the meat. Add the turkey in the Crock-Pot.

2. In the same skillet, put some extra-virgin olive oil and let it heat. Add onions and mushrooms in it. Sauté it on medium-low heat for about 6 minutes until it turns tender.

3. Put the remaining ingredients in the Crock-Pot keeping aside the cornstarch and yogurt. Cover the lid of the Crock-Pot and allow it to cook on low heat for about 4–6 hours.

4. Mix the yogurt with the cornstarch and add it to the Crock-Pot. Let it cook for about 30 minutes.

5. Serve it over brown rice.

TURKEY THIGHS IN WHITE WINE AND GARLIC

SERVING SIZE: 1
SERVINGS PER RECIPE: 6
CALORIES: 317
COOKING TIME: 4 HOURS

INGREDIENTS:

- Turkey thighs—1 ½ pounds, boneless, skin removed
- Olive oil—1 tablespoon
- Garlic cloves—6, whole
- Salt—to taste
- Lemon pepper—to taste
- Dry white wine—½ cup
- Chicken broth—½ cup
- Parsley—1 tablespoon, chopped

NUTRITION INFORMATION:

- Carbohydrate—8 g
- Protein—35 g
- Fat—14 g
- Sodium—137 mg
- Cholesterol—101 mg

INSTRUCTIONS:

1. Take the turkey in a dish and sprinkle salt and lemon pepper all over it.

2. Put a large skillet over medium-high heat. Add olive oil in it. Let it heat. Slowly add the turkey thighs in it and allow it to brown for about 10 minutes.

3. Take the Crock-Pot and place the turkey in it. Also, put the remaining ingredients in the Crock-Pot. Allow it to cook on high heat for about 3–4 hours until thoroughly cooked through.

4. Remove some of the garlic cloves from the Crock-Pot. Take the remaining garlic cloves out and mash it well. Again, put the mashed garlic cloves back into the Crock-Pot.

5. Plate the turkey on a serving dish. Pour the juice as desired.

6. Your dish is ready to be served.

CREAMY CHICKEN WITH BISCUITS

SERVING SIZE: 1
SERVINGS PER RECIPE: 6
CALORIES: 439
COOKING TIME: 6 HOURS 15 MINUTES

INGREDIENTS:

Chicken thighs—1 ½ pounds, boneless, skinless

Carrots—¾ pounds, cut into 1-inch lengths

Celery stalks—2, thinly sliced

Onion—1, small, chopped

All-purpose flour—¼ cup

Poultry seasoning—½ teaspoon

Kosher salt—to taste

Black pepper—to taste

Dry white wine—½ cup

Chicken broth—½ cup, low sodium

Easy drop biscuits—6, split

Heavy cream—½ cup

NUTRITION INFORMATION:

Carbohydrate—22 g

Protein—28 g

Fat—27 g

Sodium—911 mg

Cholesterol—95 mg

INSTRUCTIONS:

1. Take the Crock-Pot and add onion, carrots, celery, and flour in it. Toss it together. Place the chicken on top of this layer. Sprinkle poultry seasoning all over it. Sprinkle 1 teaspoon of salt and ¼ teaspoon of black pepper all over the chicken. Now add the chicken broth and dry white wine in the Crock-Pot.

2. Cover the lid of the Crock-Pot and allow it to cook on low heat for about 5–6 hours. Cook until the chicken and the vegetables are well cooked and tender. You can also cook on high heat for about 2 ½–3 hours.

3. Prepare the biscuits when 30 minutes is left before serving.

4. While it cooks, 10 minutes before it's done, add the cream and ½ teaspoon of salt in the Crock-Pot. Stir well. Cover the lid of the Crock-Pot and let it cook for 5–10 minutes more until heated through.

5. Place half of the biscuits at the bottom of the bowls. Put the chicken mixture on top of the biscuit layer. Create another layer of the remaining biscuits on top of the chicken mixture,

6. Your dish is ready to be served.

TURKEY TETRAZZINI

SERVING SIZE: 1
SERVINGS PER RECIPE: 6
CALORIES: 879
COOKING TIME: 6 HOURS

INGREDIENTS:

Hot water—1 cup

Cream of chicken soup—1 can, 10 ¾ oz., condensed

Mushrooms—1 can, 4 oz., with liquid

Cooked turkey—2 cups, diced

Cheddar cheese—1 cup, shredded

Onion—¼ cup, finely chopped

Parsley flakes—1 teaspoon, dried

Spaghetti—2 cups, broken uncooked

NUTRITION INFORMATION:

Carbohydrate—21 g

Protein—106 g

Fat—39 g

Sodium—827 mg

Cholesterol—347 mg

INSTRUCTIONS:

1. Spray the inside of the Crock-Pot with cooking spray.

2. Take a bowl and put cream of chicken soup, water, and the mushrooms along with liquid in it. Mix it well.

3. Add turkey, onion, parsley, and cheese. Stir well.

4. Now add the broken spaghetti and stir again to combine it well. Pour it into the Crock-Pot.

5. Cover the lid of the Crock-Pot and allow it to cook on low heat for about 4–6 hours until the spaghetti is well cooked and soft.

6. Stir again.

7. Your turkey tetrazzini is ready to be served.

SWEET AND SOUR CHICKEN WITH PINEAPPLE

SERVING SIZE: 1
SERVINGS PER RECIPE: 6
CALORIES: 1468
COOKING TIME: 6 HOURS

INGREDIENTS:

- Butter—4 tablespoons, melted
- White vinegar—½ cup
- Brown sugar—¾ cup
- Worcestershire sauce—3 tablespoons
- Garlic cloves—2, minced
- Salt—to taste
- Black pepper—to taste
- Red pepper flakes—as required
- Chicken broth—1 ½ cups
- Chicken breast halves—6, boneless, skinless
- Pineapple chunks—1 can, 8 oz., drained

NUTRITION INFORMATION:

- Carbohydrate—51 g
- Protein—134 g
- Fat—78 g
- Sodium—972 mg
- Cholesterol—439 mg

INSTRUCTIONS:

1. Take the Crock-Pot and add the chicken in it.

2. In a bowl, put butter, vinegar, brown sugar, minced garlic, Worcestershire sauce, red pepper flakes, salt, pepper, and chicken broth in it. Combine them well. Pour the mixture on top of the chicken in the Crock-Pot.

3. Cover the lid of the Crock-Pot and allow it to cook on low heat for about 5–7 hours until the chicken turns moist and tender.

4. Put the pineapple chunks in it and cook for another 15–20 minutes.

5. Your dish is ready to be served.

DUCK CONFIT

SERVING SIZE: 1
SERVINGS PER RECIPE: 4
CALORIES: 184
COOKING TIME: 3 HOURS

INGREDIENTS:

- Duck hindquarters—4
- Sugar—2 ½ cups
- Kosher salt—2 ½ cups
- Duck fat—14 oz.
- Extra-virgin olive oil—as desirable
- Garlic cloves—2, peeled
- Peppercorns—10, crushed
- Fresh thyme—3 sprigs

NUTRITION INFORMATION:

- Carbohydrate—0 g
- Protein—11 g
- Fat—15 g
- Sodium—121 mg
- Cholesterol—46 mg

INSTRUCTIONS:

1. Take a plastic container and put the legs in it. Combine salt and sugar together and put it inside the container. Cover the lid of the container and allow it to refrigerate overnight.

2. Rinse the duck well and let it soak in cold water for about 2 hours.

3. Drain the duck from the covered cold water and place it inside the Crock-Pot.

4. Cover the duck hindquarters with duck fat. Drizzle olive oil over the duck as needed.

5. Now add the garlic, thyme, and pepper.

6. Adjust the heat of the Crock-Pot on low setting. Allow it to cook for about 3 hours until the meat is thoroughly cooked and falls off the bone.

7. Remove the duck meat from the Crock-Pot. Pour the duck fat in a bowl. Let the duck meat and fat cool down to room temperature.

8. Your duck confit is ready to be served.

CHICKEN TAMALE DIP WITH TORTILLA CHIPS

SERVING SIZE: 1
SERVINGS PER RECIPE: 8
CALORIES: 222
COOKING TIME: 2 HOURS

INGREDIENTS:

- Cheddar—¾ cups, shredded
- Monterey Jack—½ cup, shredded
- Cream cheese—8 oz., cubed
- Garlic cloves—2, minced
- Jalapeno—½, minced
- Enchilada sauce—1 can
- Rotisserie chicken—1 cup, shredded
- Chili powder—1 tablespoon
- Kosher salt—to taste
- Freshly ground black pepper—to taste
- Fresh cilantro—chopped for garnishing
- Tortilla chips

NUTRITION INFORMATION:

- Carbohydrate—25 g
- Protein—7 g
- Fat—10 g
- Sodium—600 mg
- Cholesterol—19 mg

INSTRUCTIONS:

1. Take the Crock-Pot and add all the ingredients except the cilantro in it. Combine them well.

2. Cover the lid of the Crock-Pot and allow it to cook on low heat for about 2 hours. Keep stirring frequently. Sprinkle salt and pepper as desired.

3. Once the dip is ready, garnish it with chopped cilantro.

4. Serve it with tortilla chips.

CHICKEN ALFREDO

SERVING SIZE: 1
SERVINGS PER RECIPE: 4
CALORIES: 475
COOKING TIME: 2 ½ HOURS

INGREDIENTS:

Chicken breasts—1 lb., boneless, skinless

Butter—4 tablespoons, softened

Heavy cream—2 cups

Chicken broth—1 cup

Kosher salt—to taste

Fresh ground black pepper—to taste

Garlic powder—½ teaspoon

Italian seasoning—½ teaspoon

Rigatoni—½ lb.

Parmesan—1/3 cup, freshly grated

Fresh parsley—chopped for garnishing

NUTRITION INFORMATION:

Carbohydrate—7 g

Protein—60 g

Fat—15 g

Sodium—415 mg

Cholesterol—517 mg

INSTRUCTIONS:

1. Take the Crock-Pot and add butter, chicken, heavy cream, and chicken broth in it. Sprinkle it with salt and pepper as desired. Add garlic powder and Italian seasoning as required.

2. Allow it to cook on high heat for about 2 hours until the chicken turns tender and is thoroughly cooked through. Shred the chicken well and set it aside.

3. Add the pasta in the Crock-Pot. Also, add the parmesan in it. Allow it to cook on high heat for about 20–25 minutes until the pasta has cooked well.

4. Place the shredded chicken back into the Crock-Pot. Toss it well.

5. Transfer the chicken alfredo into bowls. Garnish it with chopped parsley.

6. Your dish is ready to be served.

LECTIN-FREE SEAFOOD RECIPES USING CROCK-POT

MANHATTAN CLAM CHOWDER

SERVING SIZE: 1
SERVINGS PER RECIPE: 4
CALORIES: 601
COOKING TIME: 8 HOURS

INGREDIENTS:

- Bacon—2 oz., 2 thick slices, sliced, diced
- Onion—1 cup, chopped
- Carrots—2, thinly sliced
- Celery ribs—3, with leaves, thinly sliced
- Fresh parsley—1 tablespoon
- Salt—1 ½ teaspoons
- Black pepper—1 dash, freshly ground
- Bay leaf—1
- Dried thyme—1 teaspoon
- Sweet potatoes—3, medium, diced
- Clams—3 cans, 6 oz., undrained, minced
- Clam juice—1 bottle, 8 oz.
- Fresh parsley—for garnishing

NUTRITION INFORMATION:

- Carbohydrate—90 g
- Protein—23 g
- Fat—17 g
- Sodium—1746 mg
- Cholesterol—28 mg

INSTRUCTIONS:

1. Take a pan and fry the bacon in it until crispy. Drain the fried bacon and transfer it to a Crock-Pot.

2. Put the remaining ingredients in the Crock-Pot and stir well.

3. Cover the lid of the Crock-Pot and allow it to cook on low heat for about 6–8 hours.

4. Garnish it with chopped fresh parsley.

5. Season it with salt and black pepper as desired.

6. Your dish is ready to be served.

LEMON AND DILL SALMON

SERVING SIZE: 1
SERVINGS PER RECIPE: 2
CALORIES: 560
COOKING TIME: 2 HOURS

INGREDIENTS:

- Salmon—2 pounds
- Garlic cloves—2, minced
- Fresh dill—1 handful
- Lemon—1, sliced
- Salt—to taste
- Black pepper—to taste
- Extra-virgin olive oil—1 teaspoon

NUTRITION INFORMATION:

- Carbohydrate—10 g
- Protein—92 g
- Fat—15 g
- Sodium—700 mg
- Cholesterol—235 mg

INSTRUCTIONS:

1. Take the Crock-Pot and spray the inside of it with cooking spray.

2. In a plate, place the salmon and drizzle olive oil all over it. Sprinkle salt and pepper as desired. Rub the salmon with garlic and fresh dill.

3. Place the salmon in the Crock-Pot.

4. Add lemon slices on top of it.

5. Allow it to cook on high heat for about 1 hour or cook on low heat for about 2 hours.

6. Your dish is ready to be served.

SEA BASS IN COCONUT CREAM SAUCE

SERVING SIZE: 1
SERVINGS PER RECIPE: 2
CALORIES: 301
COOKING TIME: 1 HOUR 30 MINUTES

INGREDIENTS:

Sea bass—1, 300–500 g

Ginger—1, cut into 2-inch pieces, thinly sliced

Coconut cream—2 cups

Fish sauce—1 tablespoon

Bok choy—4 stalks

Jalapeno peppers—3 pieces

Salt—to taste

NUTRITION INFORMATION:

Carbohydrate—7 g

Protein—30 g

Fat—18 g

Sodium—70 mg

Cholesterol—80 mg

INSTRUCTIONS:

1. Take the Crock-Pot and add coconut cream, ginger, jalapeno peppers, fish sauce, and scallions in it.

2. Place the fish on top of it.

3. Put the bok choy on top of the fish.

4. Cover the lid of the Crock-Pot and allow it to cook on high heat for about 1 ½ hours.

5. Your dish is ready to be served.

LEMON PARSLEY FISH

SERVING SIZE: 1
SERVINGS PER RECIPE: 4
CALORIES: 240
COOKING TIME: 50 MINUTES

INGREDIENTS:

- Codfish fillet—1 ½ lbs.
- Onion—½, chopped
- Parsley—2 tablespoons
- Olive oil—4 teaspoons
- Lemon—1, grated rind
- Orange—1, grated rind
- Salt—to taste
- Black pepper—to taste

NUTRITION INFORMATION:

- Carbohydrate—12 g
- Protein—33 g
- Fat—6 g
- Sodium—220 mg
- Cholesterol—80 mg

INSTRUCTIONS:

1. Take the Crock-Pot and place the grease the inside of it with cooking spray.
2. Add the fish fillet to the bottom of the Crock-Pot.
3. Place all the remaining ingredients on top of it.
4. Cover the lid of the Crock-Pot.
5. Allow it to cook on low heat for about 1 ½ hours.
6. Your dish is ready to be served.

TUNA CASSEROLE

SERVING SIZE: 1
SERVINGS PER RECIPE: 6
CALORIES: 430
COOKING TIME: 4 HOURS

INGREDIENTS:

Cream of celery soup—2 cans

Chicken broth—1/3 cup

Milk—2/3 cup

Dried parsley flakes—2 tablespoons

Tuna—2 cans, 7 oz., drained

Egg noodles—10 oz., cooked

Buttered bread crumbs—3 tablespoons

NUTRITION INFORMATION:

Carbohydrate—42 g

Protein—20 g

Fat—20 g

Sodium—791 mg

Cholesterol—62 mg

INSTRUCTIONS:

1. Take a Crock-Pot and spray the inside of it with a cooking spray.

2. In a large bowl, add cream of celery soup, chicken broth, parsley, milk, vegetables, and tuna together. Mix well. Add the cooked noodles.

3. Pour the entire mixture from the bowl into the Crock-Pot. Top it with a layer of buttered bread crumbs.

4. Cover the lid of the Crock-Pot and allow it to cook on low heat for about 4–6 hours.

5. Your tuna casserole is ready to be served.

POACHED SALMON

SERVING SIZE: 1
SERVINGS PER RECIPE: 6
CALORIES: 310
COOKING TIME: 1 HOUR 10 MINUTES

INGREDIENTS:

- Water—2 cups
- Dry white wine—1 cup
- Lemon—1, thinly sliced
- Shallot—1, thinly sliced
- Bay leaf—1
- Fresh herbs—5 sprigs
- Black peppercorns—1 teaspoon
- Kosher salt—1 teaspoon
- Salmon—2 pounds, with skin, 6 fillets
- Lemon wedges—for garnishing
- Olive oil—for serving

NUTRITION INFORMATION:

- Carbohydrate—10 g
- Protein—38 g
- Fat—9 g
- Sodium—920 mg
- Cholesterol—95 mg

INSTRUCTIONS:

1. Take the Crock-Pot and add water, lemon, wine, shallots, herbs, bay leaf, peppercorns, and salt in it. Allow it to cook on high heat for about 30 minutes.

2. Rub the salmon with salt and pepper. Place the salmon in the Crock-Pot with the skin side downwards.

3. Cover the lid of the Crock-Pot and allow it to cook on low heat for about an hour. Keep checking after 45 minutes of cooking for a desirable amount of doneness with a fork.

4. Drizzle olive oil all over the salmon. Season it with salt as preferable.

5. Garnish it with lemon wedges.

6. Your poached salmon is ready to be served.

FISH CIOPPINO

SERVING SIZE: 1
SERVINGS PER RECIPE: 6
CALORIES: 434
COOKING TIME: 5 HOURS 30 MINUTES

INGREDIENTS:

- Onion—½ cup, chopped
- Dry white wine—1 cup
- Olive oil—1/3 cup
- Garlic cloves—3, minced
- Parsley—½ cup, chopped
- Hot pepper—1, chopped
- Salt—to taste
- Black pepper—to taste
- Thyme—1 teaspoon
- Basil—2 teaspoons
- Oregano—1 teaspoon
- Paprika—½ teaspoon
- Cayenne powder—½ teaspoon
- Cod—1 fillet
- Prawns—1 dozen
- Scallops—1 dozen
- Mussels—1 dozen
- Clams—1 dozen

NUTRITION INFORMATION:

Carbohydrate—27 g

Protein—39 g

Fat—16 g

Sodium—791 mg

Cholesterol—63 mg

INSTRUCTIONS:

1. Take the Crock-Pot and add all the ingredients in it except the cod, prawns, scallops, mussels, and clams.

2. Cover the lid of the Crock-Pot and allow it to cook on low heat for about 6–8 hours.

3. When 30 minutes is left before serving, add the seafood. Adjust the heat to high heat and stir frequently.

4. Your fish cioppino is ready to be served.

CRAB RANGOON DIP

SERVING SIZE: 1
SERVINGS PER RECIPE: 4
CALORIES: 540
COOKING TIME: 45 MINUTES

INGREDIENTS:

- Cream cheese—16 oz., softened
- Sour cream—½ cup
- Green onions—4 whole, chopped
- Worcestershire sauce—1 ½ teaspoons
- Powdered sugar—2 tablespoons
- Garlic powder—½ teaspoon
- Imitation crab meat—12 oz., shredded

NUTRITION INFORMATION:

- Carbohydrate—11 g
- Protein—23 g
- Fat—45 g
- Sodium—660 mg
- Cholesterol—205 mg

INSTRUCTIONS:

1. Take the Crock-Pot and add all the ingredients in it. Stir well.

2. Cover the lid of the Crock-Pot and allow it to cook on low heat for about 2 hours.

3. Your dish is ready to be served.

GARLIC BUTTER TILAPIA

SERVING SIZE: 1
SERVINGS PER RECIPE: 4
CALORIES: 15
COOKING TIME: 45 MINUTES

INGREDIENTS:

- Tilapia fillets—4
- Garlic compound butter—2 tablespoons, chopped into small pieces
- Salt—to taste
- Pepper—to taste

NUTRITION INFORMATION:

- Carbohydrate—3 g
- Protein—1 g
- Fat—0 g
- Sodium—220 mg
- Cholesterol—0 mg

INSTRUCTIONS:

1. Take a large sheet of aluminum foil. Place the tilapia fillets in the middle and season it with salt and pepper as desired.
2. Generously divide the garlic compound butter pieces all over the fillets.
3. Wrap the fillets with the foil from all the sides.
4. Place the foil inside the Crock-Pot and cover the lid of the Crock-Pot.
5. Allow it to cook on high heat for about 2 hours.
6. Your dish is ready to be served.

BAYOU GUMBO

SERVING SIZE: 1
SERVINGS PER RECIPE: 6
CALORIES: 460
COOKING TIME: 5 HOURS

INGREDIENTS:

- Oil—3 tablespoons
- Smoked sausage—½ lb., cut into ½-inch pieces
- Frozen cut okra—2 cups
- Onion—1, large, chopped
- Garlic cloves—3, minced
- Ground red cayenne pepper—¼ teaspoon
- Flour—3 tablespoons
- Black pepper—¼ teaspoon
- Cooked shrimp—12 oz., frozen, medium, shelled, deveined, rinsed
- Long grain white rice—1 ½ cups, uncooked
- Water—3 cups

NUTRITION INFORMATION:

- Carbohydrate—47 g
- Protein—14 g
- Fat—24 g
- Sodium—640 mg
- Cholesterol—40 mg

INSTRUCTIONS:

1. In a saucepan, add oil and flour and mix them together. Cook it over medium-high heat for about 5 minutes by stirring frequently.

2. Adjust the heat to medium heat and cook for another 10 minutes until the mixture turns reddish brown in color. Keep stirring.

3. Transfer the oil and flour mixture into the Crock-Pot.

4. Add the rest of the ingredients in the Crock-Pot except the rice, shrimp, and water. Cover the lid of the Crock-Pot and allow it to cook on low heat for about 7–9 hours.

5. Meanwhile, cook the rice separately according to the package instructions.

6. Add the shrimps in the gumbo mixture and mix it well. Cover the lid of the Crock-Pot again and let it cook on low heat for another 20 minutes.

7. Take a plate and put some rice on it. Pour the gumbo over the rice.

8. Your bayou gumbo is ready to be served.

CREAMY SHRIMP AND SCALLOP SOUP

SERVING SIZE: 1
SERVINGS PER RECIPE: 6
CALORIES: 290
COOKING TIME: 3 HOURS

INGREDIENTS:

- Shrimp—1 cup, peeled, deveined
- Bay scallops—1 cup
- Onion—1, diced
- Carrot—1, large, chopped
- Butter—3 tablespoons, divided
- Flour—¼ cup
- Milk—2 cups
- Half-and-half—2 cups
- Chicken broth—¼ cup
- Thyme—1 teaspoon
- Salt—to taste
- Pepper—to taste
- Cayenne pepper—½ teaspoon

NUTRITION INFORMATION:

- Carbohydrate—17 g
- Protein—15 g
- Fat—18 g
- Sodium—330 mg
- Cholesterol—110 mg

INSTRUCTIONS:

1. Take a large saucepan and add butter in it. Add the shrimps and scallops in it. Cook until the shrimps turn pink in color and are well cooked. Transfer the scallops and shrimps to the Crock-Pot.

2. Place carrot and onion to the bottom of the Crock-Pot. Mix the seafood together with it.

3. Sprinkle flour all over it. Pour the milk, chicken broth, and half-and-half in the Crock-Pot.

4. Season it with cayenne pepper, thyme, salt, and pepper. Stir again.

5. Now add the butter in the Crock-Pot and allow it to cook on low heat for about 2–3 hours until it gains a thicker consistency.

6. Your dish is ready to be served.

TUNA SALPICAO

SERVING SIZE: 1
SERVINGS PER RECIPE: 3
CALORIES: 300
COOKING TIME: 4 HOURS

INGREDIENTS:

- Tuna loin—250 grams, cut into 1-inch cubes
- Olive oil—1 cup
- Garlic—1 whole, finely chopped
- Jalapeno peppers—4, finely chopped
- Red chili—3 pieces, finely chopped
- Black peppercorns—2 teaspoons, coarsely ground
- Salt—1 teaspoon

NUTRITION INFORMATION:

- Carbohydrate—5 g
- Protein—30 g
- Fat—17 g
- Sodium—0 mg
- Cholesterol—0 mg

INSTRUCTIONS:

1. Take the Crock-Pot and add olive oil, garlic, black peppercorns, jalapenos, red chili, and salt in it. Cover the lid of the Crock-Pot and allow it to cook on low heat for about 4 hours.

2. Adjust the temperature to high heat after sometime.

3. Add tuna in the Crock-Pot and cook for another 10 minutes.

4. Your tuna salpicao is ready to be served.

LECTIN-FREE BEEF, PORK, AND LAMB USING CROCK-POT

MONGOLIAN BEEF

SERVING SIZE: 1
SERVINGS PER RECIPE: 6
CALORIES: 593
COOKING TIME: 8 HOURS

INGREDIENTS:

- Beef chuck roast—2 lbs., fat trimmed
- Water—¼ cup
- Dark brown sugar—½ cup
- Garlic cloves—3, minced
- Ginger—2 teaspoons, minced
- Green onions—4, sliced into 2-inch pieces
- Olive oil—1 tablespoon
- Worcestershire sauce—1 tablespoon
- Cornstarch—2 tablespoons

NUTRITION INFORMATION:

- Carbohydrate—19 g
- Protein—48 g
- Fat—35 g
- Sodium—800 mg
- Cholesterol—25 mg

INSTRUCTIONS:

1. Take the Crock-Pot and add beef, water, Worcestershire sauce, garlic, brown sugar, and ginger in it. Combine them well. Allow it to cook on low heat for about 8–10 hours.

2. Shred the beef meat well and get rid of the excess fat, if any. Cover the meat to let it stay hot.

3. Take a small skillet and add 2 tablespoons of the cornstarch and 4 tablespoons of the water. Also, take out ½ cup of the cooking liquid and add it to the skillet. Whisk all of them together to gain a thick consistency. Let it heat over medium heat.

4. Pour the thickened sauce into the Crock-Pot and stir well.

5. Drizzle some of this sauce over the meat.

6. Garnish it with cooked green onions.

7. Your Mongolian beef is ready to be served.

LAMB ROAST WITH GARLIC, LEMON, AND ROSEMARY

SERVING SIZE: 1
SERVINGS PER RECIPE: 6
CALORIES: 492
COOKING TIME: 8 HOURS

INGREDIENTS:

- Leg of lamb—3 lbs.
- Garlic cloves—4, finely sliced
- Rosemary leaves—a sprig, dried
- Olive oil—as required
- Salt—to taste
- Pepper—to taste
- Lemon—1, halved

NUTRITION INFORMATION:

- Carbohydrate—0.6 g
- Protein—42 g
- Fat—34.4 g
- Sodium—129.7 mg
- Cholesterol—154.2 mg

INSTRUCTIONS:

1. Take the leg of lamb and make deep incisions on it with the help of a sharp small knife.

2. Put a piece of garlic and few rosemary leaves inside the incisions. Repeat the process with all the incisions.

3. Drizzle olive oil in small proportion all over the lamb.

4. Sprinkle salt and pepper as desired.

5. Put the lamb leg inside the Crock-Pot.

6. Now squeeze the half lemon all over the lamb leg. Leave the lemon shell at the bottom of the Crock-Pot.

7. Allow the lamb to cook on low heat for about 8–10 hours. You can also cook on high heat for about 4–5 hours. Make sure the lamb is well cooked and shreds easily.

8. Your dish is ready to be served.

LAMB CHOPS

SERVING SIZE: 2
SERVINGS PER RECIPE: 4
CALORIES: 201
COOKING TIME: 4 HOURS

INGREDIENTS:

- Onion—1, medium, sliced
- Dried oregano—1 teaspoon
- Dried thyme—½ teaspoon
- Garlic powder—½ teaspoon
- Salt—¼ teaspoon
- Pepper—1/8 teaspoon
- Lamb loin chops—1 ¾ lbs., 8
- Garlic cloves—2, minced

NUTRITION INFORMATION:

- Carbohydrate—5 g
- Protein—26 g
- Fat—8 g
- Sodium—219 mg
- Cholesterol—79 mg

INSTRUCTIONS:

1. Take the Crock-Pot and add the onion in it.

2. Place the lamb chops on a dish. Mix oregano, garlic powder, and thyme, salt, and pepper together. Rub this mix all over the lamb chops. Place the lamb chops on top of the onions in the Crock-Pot.

3. Place the garlic on top of the lamb chops.

4. Cover the lid of the Crock-Pot and allow it to cook on low heat for about 4–6 hours until the meat is well cooked and soft.

5. Your lamb chops are ready to be served.

CUBAN MOJO PORK

SERVING SIZE: 1
SERVINGS PER RECIPE: 8
CALORIES: 554
COOKING TIME: 8 HOURS

INGREDIENTS:

- Canola oil—2 tablespoons
- Kosher salt—2 teaspoons
- Black pepper—¼ teaspoon
- Pork shoulder—4 lbs.
- Orange juice—¼ cup
- Lime juice—¼ cup
- Cumin—2 teaspoons
- Dried oregano—2 teaspoons
- Red pepper flakes—¼ teaspoon, crushed
- Garlic cloves—4, minced
- Bay leaves—2
- Cornstarch—1 tablespoon
- Water—1 tablespoon

NUTRITION INFORMATION:

- Carbohydrate—4 g
- Protein—40 g
- Fat—41 g
- Sodium—260 mg
- Cholesterol—160 mg

INSTRUCTIONS:

1. Take a pot and add the canola oil in it. Let it heat on medium-high heat.

2. Sprinkle the pork with the desired amount of kosher salt and black pepper. Put the pork in the oil and allow it to brown on all the sides.

3. Take the Crock-Pot and add orange juice, cumin, lime juice, oregano, garlic, bay leaves, and red pepper flakes. Combine them well.

4. Now add them to the Crock-Pot and coat well in the mixture.

5. Allow it to cook on low heat for about 8 hours. You can also cook it on high heat for about 6 hours.

6. Add 1 tablespoon of cornstarch and 1 tablespoon of water in the Crock-Pot before the last 30 minutes. Allow it to cook on high heat for about 30 minutes to gain a thicker consistency.

7. Place the pork on a serving dish. Drizzle the thickened juice on top of it.

8. Your Cuban mojo pork is ready to be served.

BEEF AND BROCCOLI

SERVING SIZE: 1
SERVINGS PER RECIPE: 6
CALORIES: 142
COOKING TIME: 4 HOURS 20 MINUTES

INGREDIENTS:

- Sirloin steak—1 ½ lbs., thinly sliced
- Beef broth—1 cup, low sodium
- Brown sugar—½ cup
- Sesame oil—3 tablespoons
- Sriracha—1 tablespoon
- Garlic cloves—3, minced
- Green onions—3, thinly sliced
- Cornstarch—2 tablespoons
- Broccoli florets—2 cups
- Sesame seeds—for garnishing
- Green onions—for garnishing

NUTRITION INFORMATION:

- Carbohydrate—12 g
- Protein—7 g
- Fat—13 g
- Sodium—710 mg
- Cholesterol—10 mg

INSTRUCTIONS:

1. Take a Crock-Pot and add the steak in it. Put the beef broth, brown sugar, sesame oil, garlic, green onions, and sriracha in it.

2. Cover the lid of the Crock-Pot and allow it to cook on low heat for about 3 ½–4 hours. Make sure the beef is thoroughly cooked and turns tender too.

3. In a bowl, add the cornstarch and few tablespoons of the cooking broth in it. Whisk it well.

4. Add the cornstarch mixture in the Crock-Pot and toss the beef well until it is fully combined. Put the broccoli florets in the Crock-Pot and allow it to cook covered for about 20 minutes or more.

5. Garnish it with sesame seeds and sliced green onions.

6. Your dish is ready to be served.

IRISH LAMB STEW

SERVING SIZE: 1
SERVINGS PER RECIPE: 8
CALORIES: 247
COOKING TIME: 8 HOURS

INGREDIENTS:

- Leg of lamb—2 lbs., boneless, trimmed, cut into 1-inch pieces
- Sweet potatoes—1 ¾ lbs., peeled, cut into 1-inch pieces
- Leeks—3, large, white part only, halved, thinly sliced
- Carrots—3, large, peeled, cut into 1-inch pieces
- Celery stalks—3, thinly sliced
- Chicken broth—1 can, 14 oz., reduced sodium
- Fresh thyme—2 teaspoons, chopped
- Salt—1 teaspoon
- Freshly ground pepper—1 teaspoon
- Fresh parsley leaves—¼ cup, chopped

NUTRITION INFORMATION:

- Carbohydrate—26 g
- Protein—21 g
- Fat—6 g
- Sodium—499 mg
- Cholesterol—58 mg

INSTRUCTIONS:

1. Take a Crock-Pot and add lamb, leeks, carrots, thyme, celery, chicken broth, salt, and pepper in it. Stir well. Cover the lid of the Crock-Pot and allow it to cook on low heat for about 8 hours until the lamb is tender.

2. Add parsley to the Crock-Pot. Stir again.

3. Your Irish lamb stew is ready to be served.

CREAMY RANCH PORK CHOPS

SERVING SIZE: 1
SERVINGS PER RECIPE: 4
CALORIES: 330
COOKING TIME: 5 HOURS

INGREDIENTS:

Bone-in pork loin chops—2 lbs., 4

Ranch dressing and seasoning mix—1 package, 1 oz.

Creamy mushroom soup—1 can, 18 oz.

Cornstarch—2 tablespoons

NUTRITION INFORMATION:

Carbohydrate—13 g

Protein—35 g

Fat—16 g

Sodium—1100 mg

Cholesterol—95 mg

INSTRUCTIONS:

1. Take the Crock-Pot and spray the inside of it with a cooking spray.

2. Season the pork with ranch dressing mix on both the sides.

3. Put the pork chops in the Crock-Pot and pour the creamy mushroom soup all over it.

4. Cover the lid of the Crock-Pot and allow it to cook for about 5–6 hours on low heat until tender. Take the pork chops out from the Crock-Pot and keep them aside.

5. Take a small bowl and add cornstarch and water in it. Whisk it well. Add the cornstarch mixture into the creamy mushroom sauce inside the Crock-Pot. Continue cooking on low heat for about 3–5 minutes. Make sure the sauce gains a thicker consistency.

6. Pour it over the pork chops.

7. Your dish is ready to be served.

ITALIAN BEEF

SERVING SIZE: 1
SERVINGS PER RECIPE: 8
CALORIES: 288
COOKING TIME: 6 HOURS

INGREDIENTS:

Beef chuck roast—3 lbs.

Red onion—1, large, sliced

Garlic cloves—5, minced

Pepperoncinis—15

Butter—4 tablespoons

Red wine—½ cup

Worcestershire sauce—¼ cup

Brown sugar—3 tablespoons

Italian seasoning—1 tablespoon, dried

Red pepper flakes—¼ teaspoon, crushed

NUTRITION INFORMATION:

Carbohydrate—2 g

Protein—42 g

Fat—11 g

Sodium—216 mg

Cholesterol—124 mg

INSTRUCTIONS:

1. Take the Crock-Pot and place the beef roast at the bottom of it. Put the remaining ingredients on top of the beef roast.

2. Cover the lid of the Crock-Pot and allow it to cook on high heat for about 4–6 hours. You can also cook on low heat for about 8–10 hours.

3. The beef should be well cooked and tender. Shred the beef meat with the help of two forks. The shredded meat should be well absorbed in the juice.

4. Your Italian beef is ready to be served.

MOROCCAN LAMB

SERVING SIZE: 1
SERVINGS PER RECIPE: 4
CALORIES: 358
COOKING TIME: 4 HOURS

INGREDIENTS:

- Lamb chops—2 lbs.
- Moroccan spice rub—2 tablespoons
- Carrots—¼ lb., chopped
- Onion—¼ cup, sliced
- Fresh mint—¼ cup, chopped
- Chicken broth—¼ cup, low sodium

NUTRITION INFORMATION:

- Carbohydrate—6.7 g
- Protein—45.4 g
- Fat—15.6 g
- Sodium—184.4 mg
- Cholesterol—149.7 mg

INSTRUCTIONS:

1. Take the Crock-Pot and pour the chicken broth into the bottom of it.
2. Place the lamb meat on a plate and rub 2 tablespoons of the spice rub all over the lamb.
3. Put the lamb meat and the vegetables in the Crock-Pot.
4. Garnish it with fresh mint. Allow it to cook on high heat for about 3–4 hours. You can also cook it on low heat for about 6–8 hours.
5. Your Moroccan lamb is ready to be served.

GINGER BEEF

SERVING SIZE: 1
SERVINGS PER RECIPE: 6
CALORIES: 230
COOKING TIME: 8 HOURS

INGREDIENTS:

- Beef roast—2 lbs., cut into 1-inch cubes
- Carrots—3, cut into 1-inch thick slices
- Scallions—1 cup, sliced
- Garlic cloves—3, minced
- Fresh ginger—4 tablespoons, grated
- Beef stock—1 ½ cups
- Tamari sauce—2 tablespoons
- Red pepper flakes—1 teaspoon
- Tapioca—2 tablespoons
- Salt—1 teaspoon
- Pepper—½ teaspoon

NUTRITION INFORMATION:

- Carbohydrate—10 g
- Protein—28 g
- Fat—9 g
- Sodium—525 mg
- Cholesterol—0 mg

INSTRUCTIONS:

1. Take the Crock-Pot and add all the ingredients in it.

2. Cover the lid of the Crock-Pot and allow it to cook on low heat for about 6–8 hours. You can also cook on high heat for about 3–4 hours.

3. Your ginger beef is ready to be served.

BRAISED LAMB SHANKS WITH ROSEMARY AND MUSHROOMS

SERVING SIZE: 1
SERVINGS PER RECIPE: 4
CALORIES: 400
COOKING TIME: 2 ½ HOURS

INGREDIENTS:

- Olive oil—½ tablespoon

- Lamb shanks—4, fat trimmed

- Carrots—2, peeled, diced

- Celery stalk—3, diced

- Onion—½, diced

- Cremini mushrooms—500 g, stems removed

- Garlic cloves—2, sliced

- Red wine—¾ cup

- Beef stock—¾ cup, fat reduced

- Mustard—2 tablespoons

- Bay leaf—1

- Rosemary—1 ½ tablespoons, minced

- Orange—rind of ½ large

- Balsamic vinegar—1 tablespoon

NUTRITION INFORMATION:

Carbohydrate—11 g

Protein—49 g

Fat—17 g

Sodium—345 mg

Cholesterol—145 mg

INSTRUCTIONS:

1. Take a large skillet and add oil in it. Let the oil get preheated over medium-high heat.

2. Sprinkle the lamb shanks with pepper and salt. Let it brown on all the sides.

3. Place the lamb shanks in the Crock-Pot.

4. Add onion, carrots, and celery in the pan and sauté it for about 5–7 minutes. Put the mushrooms and garlic in it. Stir again.

5. Pour wine in the pan and allow it to deglaze. Scrape out all the bits stuck to the pan. Transfer the entire thing to the Crock-Pot and also add beef stock, bay leaf, mustard, orange rind, and rosemary. Allow it to cook on high heat for about 6 hours.

6. Add the vinegar before serving. Stir well. Sprinkle salt and pepper as desired. Discard the visible excess fat from the sauce surface.

7. Your dish is ready to be served.

ABOUT THE AUTHOR

Mellisa Armstrong is a health and fitness enthusiast who loves teaching people about healthy ways to lose weight and live the best life they can.

Over the years, she has studied what works and what doesn't in health and fitness. She is passionate about helping others achieve great success in their diet and exercise endeavor through her books and seminars.

Her biggest satisfaction is when she finds out that she was able to help someone attain the results they've been looking for. In her free time, she loves to spend time with her 2-year-old daughter.

Printed in Great Britain
by Amazon